Physics

AF711783

Biology

Biochemistry

Psychology

Copyright

Table of Contents

General Chemistry

Organic Chemistry

Sociology

Author's Note

If you are reading this, you're brave. You have decided to attack a quintessential exam: the MCAT. The exam is tough, broad, and unforgiving for 7½ hours (with a few stress breaks in between). You are committed to getting the highest score you can for that coveted med. school admission.

Whether your exam is a few years or a few months away, we at Cambridge 10 have been there with you all. Most of us are pre-meds, ex-med-schoolers and doctors. Most of us took the MCAT multiple times just to make this book! Either way, we understand one fundamental fact. It is an illusion that anyone who takes this well prepared. Whether you studied for 2 weeks or 2 years in advance, everyone gets hit with some curve-balls no matter how many practice questions, flashcards, or expensive courses you've taken.

What we realized after every hopeless 10+ hour study day and all the exam room anxiety is the following. No one needs yet another test prep book with 700 reworded practice questions. No one needs tips like "eat a granola bar!", "make sure to bring water!" In short, no one needs something the regurgitated study tips, or 20-year-old notes, or another time-sink that only makes your studies more difficult. If your serious about this test, you have enough of those challenges already. Instead, we realized that we needed, in addition to the practice test, question banks, and so on... Something that shortcuts the long path to learning--that builds new connections that save us time and energy. And lastly, that allows some creativity and positivity amidst the sleepless, draining study nights.

Thus, this book is about solving one problem and one problem only: how to keep that god-almighty massive amount of information in our tiny little brains to win at this exam. No deep critical thinking here, just quick memory shortcuts that allow our prefrontal cortex to live to fight another day. *This* is the key. A small shortcut, a small optimization that adds up, saving in the end lots of time and mental energy. This is simple breakthrough we figured out after we testing dozens of ideas. After refining a study and memory strategy and developing on aspiring med-schoolers of all backgrounds, we had a blueprint to get little knowledge and preparation to 513 and above on the MCAT.

Let us be clear, the path we take in this book is *not* a silver bullet that effortlessly gets you that magic number you envision on your score report. The process we outline requires intentionality, creativity, and awareness even... No *especially* on study days you feel most exhausted. We can't offer magic, but we can offer a foundation that has been battle-tested by many, us included, that you can build on through discipline and creativity to accelerate your score improvement.

On the flip side, our key strategy of remembering and personalizing your own mnemonics can be fun and creative aspect of your studies... A break from the drudgery of critically thinking to anxiously converge on an answer on your 700th practice test. In fact, the best mnemonics are like little mind viruses. They are created by you and only to benefit you. They can be right there when you need them many years later when you've secured your dream, and want nothing to do with the MCAT ever again.

So, we hope to have convinced you a little on how underrated mnemonics really are. This is *the* important belief you need going into the MCAT. It allows you to buy into storing mnemonics in a brain that initially wants to forget it. This belief allows you to creatively generate mnemonics, to visualize them, to create a story for them, to place them in your unique mind. The specific testing-backed strategies and research-supported processes for implementing these memory tricks in your study we will discuss in the next section **How to Use**.

Overall, this is a deceptively simple book... An index of some good mnemonics. But, it is up to you to adopt our tried-and-tested study process. You will need to fill in the blanks--to buy into creating a memory system that saves mental effort for the questions/sections that matter most... The differ ence maker for a higher score. For this reason we provide specific strategies and outline a study process that incorporates this book with others to maximizes your success. The mental tricks in this book, and those that you write on your own, should offset the pain of having that TCA enzyme on the tip of your tongue and missing out on big points because of it. We hope you can use these tools to succeed.

We hope you enjoy this book. If you found it at all useful please leave us a ★★★★★ wherever you found us. If you have any feedback on how to improve, email us at support@cambridgeten.com. We are a small startup team of students and professionals with a mission **to give ambitious people real strategies to help them succeed on any exam**.

If you are interested in a complete exam study platform, **sign up and create a study plan at cambridgeten.com**. The coupon below gets you 20% off a monthly subscription! You can also sign up for our MCAT tips email newsletter. If you notice errors in the book, email us , and whenever we update it we will send you a free updated e-book copy and refund your test prep subscription. Thanks for reading. We're rooting for you!

Sincerely,

The Cambridge Ten Team

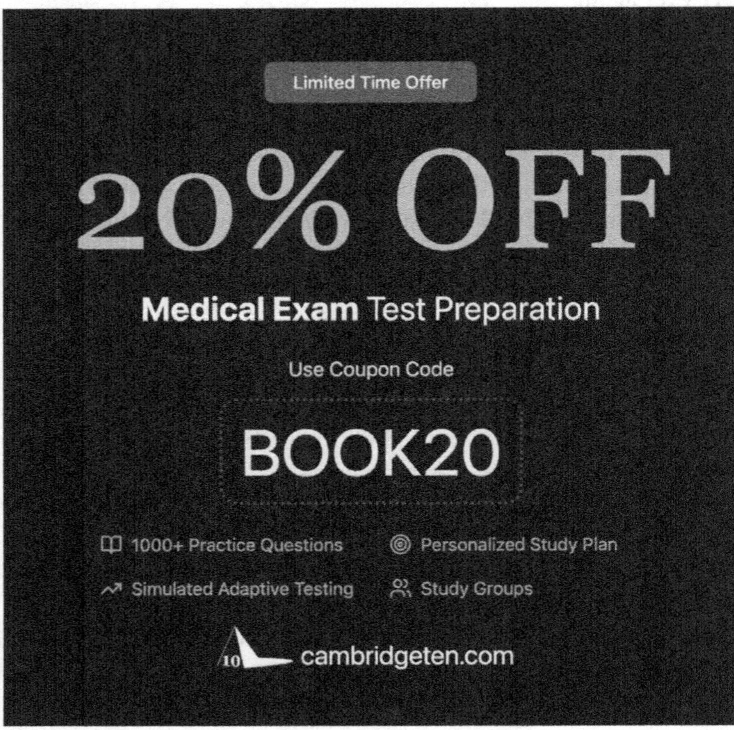

How to Use

What is this book?

This book is an index of the most popular an effective mnemonics for the MCAT exam. It is split up into topic sections, but the topics are still connected for use in order of the test: Chemistry/Physics, then Biology/Biochem, then last Psychology/Sociology. We will used the shortened acronyms to refer to each: **C/P, B/B, P/S**. This book is meant to be flipped through as you study and do practice tests so you can easily search for something you need.

The Blank Pages, Make Your Own

The blank pages at the end of each section are meant for you to fill in, add your own mnemonics, write down group-study notes, etc. They should be related to the mnemonic on the right, even if only tangentially. Let's run through some examples:

- *"the mnemonic for this sucks! I have my own!"*: This is great! Feel free to get a giant marker and scribble out our entire page and write your mnemonic down on the blank page. In fact, we find many do this for memorable vulgar mnemonics (... we just don't want to be canceled)

- *"I want to write a little cheat sheet for questions/topics related to this mnemonic"*: This is useful, but understand that simplicity is key. Cramming all the information onto a single page like you do for college exams won't work well. Our strategy is to create more shortcuts for your brain to remember as opposed to spend mental energy. For this reason, we recommend making sure the content is a mnemonic, rhyme, ordered list, drawing, etc. Anything that has a well defined pattern, emotional connection, visualization, or all of those at the same time.

- *"I don't care about your system, I'll write whatever I want!"*: Thats totally OK. After all, these are just guide lines, not a double-blind randomized controlled trial. No matter what you want to do, remember to be aware if it is working for you, otherwise cut it. For example, we found that students that created a **5 Principle Study Plan** (in the next section) were more committed and more positive throughout the study and test-taking process. So... if you end up not using this book, thats alright! As long as you take-away that the path to success is you putting that systematic effort in even under stress and constraint. That is what we believe will train you to stay diligent and positive on the long road to MCAT success.

So, I hope you understand the importance of these blank pages. Remember that it doesn't have to be perfect. In fact, most students we tested wrote on less than half of the blank pages. However, those that wrote at least 1 or 2 small things on at least 30% of the blank pages tended to perform significantly better than the others. As you take on your study, primarily when you are doing content review, take advantage of developing your internal bank of mnemonics early and often. The more questions on which you recall the mnemonic, even when not related to the answering the question, allows it to transfer into long-term memory.

The Study Plan

Now that we have understood how to use this book and even populate it with our own memory tricks, let's look at testing strategy. These are strategies we have tested extensively by running MCAT tutoring programs for students of all backgrounds.

First, once you have selected your test-date, reverse engineer your schedule. What time commitments do you have? School? Work? Personal time? You need 200 hours of studying *minimum*, so do the math and see how many hours each day or week you can study given your respective time commitments. If the math isn't adding up, you will unfortunately need to make a sacrifice (even if it is for more personal time to rest and rejuvenate). Now, as soon as possible, it's time to take your first practice test.

Practice Test 1: Your first practice test should establish a baseline. Timed. No studying. No content review or questions. All the practice tests you do should be serious and replicate a testing environment to the best of your ability and resources. Even simply eating the same snacks on your breaks, wearing similar clothing, having fine-point marker will be an asset come test day. Now, why do a practice test before any studying? Consider you study a bunch then take your first test, then study some more and take a second. How would you feel if the second score was lower than your first? We've seen many smart, diligent self-studying students make this basic mistake and suddenly so lose so much morale. Studying for the MCAT is a marathon, and we need all the morale we can get! So put your ego of a low score away. Instead, set a baseline so that your score, no matter how low, gives you faith you will only go onward and upward! The score isn't the brag. The change in score is.

High Content Phase: Now it's time to dive into the content. This phase is the first half of your study plan duration. Here you need to focus 80% on content and 20% on practice (in the next phase, these will flip). We recommend creating an Excel table of all chapters of all the books you have procured to use covering all subjects. While online courses/content can be useful, we still recommend books to get in the habit of annotating, writing mnemonics, and other tactile methods to engage memory and actually use the noteboard booklet during the exam. Based on our testing, here are more strategies to consider:

- Go through each book/subject in parallel. This makes sure you don't forget the initial subject and continue to retain information and mnemonic connections.

- CARS will be a consistent task you do every day. 1-3 passages each day. CARS is a quarter of your score whether you like it or not, and certain medical schools prioritize this score over all others. Do a passage (via AAMC Question Packs) followed by careful analysis of your responses, rereading often. This will guarantee you are building the intuition to improve your CARS score.

- Alternate between easy and hard days. This can even be subject dependent. Eg. spend one day for a biochem. deep dive, then the next day going through 1-2 short physics topics. Eg. spend one day doing stressful timed B/B sections, then the next day doing an interesting psych. topic.

- Be diligent about the work. This exam rewards breadth of applicable knowledge... so you need to apply all the knowledge available. This is the make-or-break phase where good study skills and time-management form and shine. You will be enticed to add "just another week" to catch up, but this is a cartoonishly slippery slope that we've seen many fall behind on. If you need to update your plan, update early and be honest with yourself. Commit to the dates, and reward yourself at the end of the day or on an off-day for sticking to the program.

Practice Test 2-3: These should be taken early during the High Content Phase. These are extremely important as they are the two early feedback mechanisms that highlight what content to focus on (and the depth of knowledge you may honestly be lacking in specific topics). After taking test, take the next day off. We recommend taking it Saturday, and a break on Sunday... but this is at the discretion of your schedule.

High Practice Phase: This will be the latter half of your study plan duration: 80% practice 20% content. At this point you will mostly be taking practice exams/sections and reviewing content you missed (for example question topics that you missed in earlier practice exams). Remember: every step of the feedback loop is important. You will be tempted to calculate your score and move on, when in fact you should be deep diving on the questions you got wrong. You need to be level-headed. You a physics major but missed a bunch of optics questions? Don't discount them as silly mistakes or worse beat yourself up over them. Just go back and quickly review the topics, watch some videos, etc. Understand down to atomic detail why you didn't get that question by perpetually asking why (even if the deeper answer is something embarrassing like "*I didn't read this part because I was distracted by thinking about a question I didn't get last passage*"). We have seen many-a-pre-med convince themselves that they don't need to review some specific topic, or lose morale from not getting a question they "*should*" have gotten because of X research or Y experience. It's okay to fail, this is a system, and to win we need to control our emotions. Here are some additional guidelines for this phase:

By the end of this phase, you should at a *minimum* have gone through all AAMC resources once.

Turn up the CARS practice: 3-4 passages a day. AAMC CARS Question Packs will typically be enough, but get more resources if you have a longer study timeline.

Practice Test 4-5: These should be taken during the High Practice Phase, and you can take more if you want, just don't take any the week-ish before your exam. Also, remember that a full-length is just a diagnostic tool. While test 2-3 was about finding larger subject areas you needed to focus on, 4-5 is for fine-tuning. Find more specific topics you aren't doing well on. Look for topics you aren't having success on across practice tests too (if you are doing 5 or more practice tests we recommend a Excel sheet where you keep track of missed questions by problem topic).

Once it is a week from test day, no more practice tests or passages. Instead, prioritize reviewing strong content areas so they are fresh. Take a rest day or two, doing some light work if you want. No matter how you feel about your preparation, execution, etc... you deserve to relax and de-stress so you can be successful on the big day.

Test Day Tips

Sleep, sleep, sleep: If you take away anything, get to bed early the night before (earlier than you usually do). We do not care if you can "survive on 4" or want to do some last minute review... Go to bed. If you are having trouble use supplements or prescribed medication that you have used consistently before. Do not be testing anything new the night before.

- **Be prepared, obviously:** The night before, put out clothes that you generally wore during your studying and practice exams, phone, water, ear-plugs, snacks and whatever else you need. For snacks, we recommend healthy snacks/sandwiches and a treat for when you finish the exam.

- **Use every break:** You are not cool for not taking a break. Use the bathroom, eat some food. Even a simple location change for no particular reason can allow you to better reset for the next section.

- **When it's done, it's done:** Once the exam is over, relax. Thinking over what you got right or wrong should last less than 5 minutes. After that it's over. Have a treat if you brought one, or get a treat or reward from somewhere. You deserve it!

How Does This Book Fit Into Your Plan?

Now that we have outlined a bulletproof template to your MCAT studies, let's see how this book can fit in to this template and why. Note: these are how we observed the book used among top scorers and high-improving students.

Insight #1: Use this book as an index for timed practice sections

We have tested the use of mnemonics in many forms. We unexpectedly found that a book is more useful than we thought. Why? If you use it in practice, flipping through pages quickly, you can find and reinforce your memory of mnemonics you need to answer questions. Thus, we recommend using this during timed practice sections in your everyday practice. We do not recommend doing this on practice tests, only practice passages/sections. Practice tests should be closed-source so you can accurately gauge how you are performing and pat yourself on the back for making improvements under real test conditions.

Nevertheless, while doing the timed practice passages try to recall mnemonics yourself. Write down any you think of as soon as you have skimmed a passage and determined pertinent topics. If you can't think of any, quickly flip through this book to see if any of them are relevant. If you are stuck on a *specific* question trying to recall specific information, also flip through this book. If you can't find any, note this question down. Once done with a passage and grading, look at the explanation of answers (if you have them). If you marked down the question already, or feel like you made a simple, silly mistake as you read the explanation, chances are this is where a simple mnemonic or memory tool could have helped you.

So, use a blank page in the book to brainstorm something memorable. If you feel like the explanation proved you made a more complex mistake, this should be a signal do look back at your content/research, and see if you can also make a mnemonic related to information (this is because the pain of that bigger mistake can influence you to recall memory even better the next time, given you still do some content review like we said earlier). We have also found that some students altered their study strategy, doing content for one topic but practice passages for the topic they studied yesterday, giving them a buffer to see if they could recall mnemonics well. Try this strategy and see if it works for you.

Insight #2: Take the book everywhere, if you can

This is fairly necessary if you are studying for this exam under a relatively busy schedule. If you have a full-time job with low workload or free time, than this should be mandatory. A lot of people who succeed under these circumstances especially need to siphon free time and bring portable study materials: this book, flashcards, notes, etc. Then, do practice questions on a phone/tablet.

Insight #3: Abuse every page

This is less common among people who used this book, but those who did had the most positive impact on their score and their outlook towards using the book. For example, successful students actively scribbled or even ripped out pages they didn't need, wrote and thought about more personalized mnemonics and compiled them within this book. The people who put in effort here reaped the most benefits. Even those who used the mnemonics here and merely copied them into flashcards did well (however be systematic about this and don't let the deck get too long).

The Ultimate Goal

We hope that you have found our study plan template, as well as how to use this book within that plan helpful. Our realization is that there is a simple, criminally underrated strategy that allows us to game the MCAT into getting a higher score. It's simple: this test is always a memory game first, and critical thinking right after. If we simply allocate more time to building the right encyclopedia of memory shortcuts, we can save the time it takes to recall specific information and allocate time to questions that require more mental effort. It can even be fun, light practice that you can do in the downtime of a busy schedule where you can't go hardcore-library-study-mode. The goal is to treat your brain like an emotional computer. As you prepare, you allow yourself to search for mnemonics or memory tools you have strong meaning or emotions attached to. This key unlocks further memory tools on the blank pages, so you have a population of memory tricks around which to attack each question, passage, and section. It's not easy. It's never perfect. But in the long-run, from the MCAT and beyond, you will notice the difference.

Next Tasks

Now that you have an idea about a study plan and how this book could be useful as you study for the MCAT, we recommend some basic planning and reflection strategies. First, come up with a **5 Principle Study Plan**. It should not be as specific as we described earlier, that will require proper organization and scheduling tools (but you can write specific notes on the next page. As you take your practice tests, we also recommend **Reflections** after each to distill weaknesses, reflect on your emotions, and keep yourself aware and accountable. Let's go.

5 Principle Study Plan

1.

2.

3.

4.

5

Tip: Write in pencil so you can make small refinements later! Another tip: If you are anxious to start and tend to overwork yourself, make your 5th principle about how you will **rest**. If you are a little depressed about the prospect of starting and tend to procrastinate, give yourself some kind words on how/why you will **commit** to the study plan.

✎ Additional Plan Notes:

Reflections

After Practice Test 1:

After Practice Test 2:

Reflections

After Practice Test 3:

After Practice Test 4:

After Practice Test 5:

Physics Cheat Sheet

Kinematics + Dynamics

Newton's 2nd law	$F = ma$	
Gravitational force (2 objects)	$F_g = G(m_1m_2/r^2)$	$F_g = mg$ $(\parallel = \cos\theta \perp = \sin\theta)$
Translational motion	$x = x_o + v_ot + 1/2at^2$ $(V_f)^2 = (V_o)^2 + 2ax$	$V_f = V_o + at$
Friction Force (static, kinetic)	$F_{max} = \mu N$	$\mu_k < \mu_s$ always
Uniform circular motion*	$F_c = ma_c = mv^2/r$	$a_c = v^2/r$
Momentum, Impulse*	$I = F\Delta t = \Delta M$	$M = mv$
Centripetal Force	$Fc = mv^2/r$ $(v = 2\pi r/t)$	
Torque forces	$T = rF\sin\theta$	$L_1 = F_1 \times r_1$ (CCW + ve) $L_2 = F_2 \times r_2$ (CW - ve)
Torque force at EQ	$\Sigma F_x = 0$ and $\Sigma F_y = 0$	$\Sigma L = 0$
Uniform circular motion	$F_c = ma_c = mv^2/r$	$a_c = v^2/r$
Momentum, Impulse*	$I = F\Delta t = \Delta M$	$M = mv$
Friction Force (static, kinetic)	$F_{max} = \mu N$	$\mu_k < \mu_s$ always

Work + Energy

Work ($J = kg\ m^2/s^2$), Power (Watt = J/s)	$W = Fd$	$P = \Delta W/\Delta t$
Work (additional)	$W = \Delta KE$ $(KE = 1/2mv^2)$	$W = P\Delta V$
Energy (conservation)	$E_T = E_k + E_p$	$E = mc^2$ (photon: $E = hf$)
Gravitational, Elastic Potential Energy	$U = mgh$	$U = kx^2/2$
Spring Force, Work Done by Spring	$F = -kx$	$W = kx^2/2$

Thermodynamics

Change in Internal Energy	$\Delta U = Q - W$	
Heat, Heat (phase change)	$Q = mc\Delta T$ (MCAT!)	$Q = mL$ ($\Delta T = 0$; $L = \Delta H$)
Gibbs Free Energy	$\Delta G = \Delta H - T\Delta S$	$\Delta G° = -RT\ln K_{eq}$

Electrostatics + Magnetism

Coulomb's Law, Magnitude of Elec. Field	$F_c = Kq_1q_2/r^2$	$E = F^f/q = KQ/r^2$ *(N/C)*
Electric PE, Potential	$U = kQq/r$	$V = U/q = KQ/r$ **(J/C)**
Force on moving charge, on current-carrying wire	$F_B = qvB\sin\theta$	$F_B = ILB\sin\theta$
Magnetic Force	$F_B = qvB\sin\theta$	$1\ T = 1\ N \cdot s/m \cdot C$
Lorentz Force	$F = qE + qvB\sin\theta$	

Circuits

Current and Resistance	$I = Q/t$	$R = \rho l/A$ (Ohm's: $V = IR$)
Resistors (series, parallel)	$R_s = R_1 + R_2 + \ldots$	$1/R_p = 1/R_1 + 1/R_2 + \ldots$
Capacitors series, parallel)	$1/C_s = 1/C_1 +$ $1/C_2 + 1/C_3 \ldots$	$C_p = C_1 + C_2 \ldots$
Capacitance, Capacitor PE	$C = Q/V$ *(F=C/V)*	$U = CV^2/2 = QV/2$ $= Q^2/2C$
Kirchoff's Laws	$\Sigma i = 0$ at a junction	$\Sigma\Delta V = 0$ in a loop

Fluids

Density, Weight (buoy)	$\rho = m/V$	$R = \rho l/A$ (Ohm's: $V = IR$)
Pressure, Hydrostatic Pressure	$P = F/A$	$1/R_p = 1/R_1 + 1/R_2 + \ldots$
Pascal's Principle	$P = F_1/A_1 = F_2/A_2$	$C_p = C_1 + C_2 \ldots$
Flow Rate (Poiseville, Continuity)	$Q = \pi r^4 \Delta P / (8L\mu)$	$Q = A_1 v_1 = A_2 v_2$
Bernoulli Equation	$P_1 + \rho v_1^2 + \rho g h_1 = P_2 + \rho v_2^2 + \rho g h^2$	

Waves + Sound

Wave Propagation Speed, Period	$v_p = f\lambda$	$T = 1/f$
Sound	$dB = 10 \log_{10}(I/I_0)$	beats = Δf; $I = P/A$ *(Watts/m2)*
Doppler Effect	$f' = f\,(v \pm v_0) / (v \mp v_s)$	
Harmonics open pipes, closed pipes	$\lambda = 2L/(\#\ \text{nodes})$	$\lambda = 2L/(\#\ \text{wavelengths}/4)$

Light + Optics

Speed of Light	$c = f\lambda$	$c = 299{,}792{,}458$ m/s
Refraction (Snell's)	$(\sin\theta_1)/(\sin\theta_2) = v_1/v_2 = n_2/n_1 = \lambda_1/\lambda_2$	$n = c/v$;
Thin Len's Equation, Magnification	$1/f = 1/o + 1/i = 2/r$	$m = -i/o$ *($i>0 \rightarrow$ real; $m>0 \rightarrow$ upright; $\theta>0 \rightarrow$ in-front(mirror) / same-side(lens))*
Series of Lenses (focal length, power, mag.)	$1/f = 1/f_1 + 1/f_2 + \ldots$ $P = P_1 + P_2 + \ldots$	$m = m_1 \bullet m_2 \bullet \ldots$

Tip: As you read through a physics problem, make a quick table of the knowns and unknowns (quantities to solve for) by ***symbol***. This helps jog your memory of equations you can plug in.

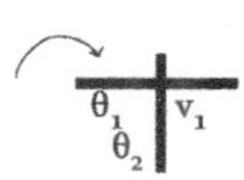

Chemistry Cheat Sheet

Group → / Period ↓	1	2	3	4	5	6	7	8	9	10	11	12	13	14	15	16	17	18
1	1 H																	2 He
2	3 Li	4 Be											5 B	6 C	7 N	8 O	9 F	10 Ne
3	11 Na	12 Mg											13 Al	14 Si	15 P	16 S	17 Cl	18 Ar
4	19 K	20 Ca	21 Sc	22 Ti	23 V	24 Cr	25 Mn	26 Fe	27 Co	28 Ni	29 Cu	30 Zn	31 Ga	32 Ge	33 As	34 Se	35 Br	36 Kr
5	37 Rb	38 Sr	39 Y	40 Zr	41 Nb	42 Mo	43 Tc	44 Ru	45 Rh	46 Pd	47 Ag	48 Cd	49 In	50 Sn	51 Sb	52 Te	53 I	54 Xe
6	55 Cs	56 Ba	* 71 Lu	72 Hf	73 Ta	74 W	75 Re	76 Os	77 Ir	78 Pt	79 Au	80 Hg	81 Tl	82 Pb	83 Bi	84 Po	85 At	86 Rn
7	87 Fr	88 Ra	** 103 Lr	104 Rf	105 Db	106 Sg	107 Bh	108 Hs	109 Mt	110 Ds	111 Rg	112 Cn	113 Nh	114 Fl	115 Mc	116 Lv	117 Ts	118 Og
			* 57 La	58 Ce	59 Pr	60 Nd	61 Pm	62 Sm	63 Eu	64 Gd	65 Tb	66 Dy	67 Ho	68 Er	69 Tm	70 Yb		
			** 89 Ac	90 Th	91 Pa	92 U	93 Np	94 Pu	95 Am	96 Cm	97 Bk	98 Cf	99 Es	100 Fm	101 Md	102 No		

Kinetics

Rate Law	rate = $k[A]^x[B]^y$	0: $[A] = [A]_0 - kt$ *(M/s)* 1: $[A] = [A]_0 e^{-kt}$ *(1/s)* 2: $1/[A] = 1/[A]_0 + kt$ *(1/Ms)*
Arhennius Eqn.	$k = Ae^{-E_a/RT}$	
Law of Mass Action	$k_{eq} = [C]^c[D]^d / [A]^a[B]^b$	

Solutions

pH; pOH	$-\log[H^+]$	$-\log[OH^-]$
Dissociation Constant (acid, base)	$K_a = [H_3O^+][A^-]/[HA]$	$Kb = [B^+][OH^-]/[BOH]$
pK_a; pK_b	$-\log K_a$	$-\log K_b$
Buffer Solution pH	$pH = pK_a +$ log [conj. base] / [acid]	$pH = pK_a = 14 - pK_b$
Solubility Product Constant	for A_mB_n: $K_{sp} = [A^{n+}]^m[B^{m-}]^n$	
Autoionization of water	$K_w = H_3O^+][OH^-] = 10^{-14}$	

Misc.

Retardation Factor	R_f = dist. spot moved / dist. solvent moved	
Henry's Law	$[A] = K_H \times P_A$	
Electrophoresis	$v = Ez/f$	→ migration velocity of molecule
Hardy-Weinberg	$(p + q)^2 = p^2+2pq + q^2 = 1$	$p + q = 1$
Michaelis-Menten	$v = v_{max} [S] / (K_m + [S])$	
Nernst Equation	$E_{cell} = E°_{cell} - (RT/nF) \ln Q$	
Osmotic Pressure	$\Pi = iMRT$	

Chapter 2

General Chemistry

H Bonding Elements

i've Had eNOF!

H	Hydrogen bonds with
N	Nitrogen
O	Oxygen
F	Fluoride

Hydroen bonding only occurs with these highly electronegative atoms since they have enough power to attract the hydrogen electron to form a bond

Electronegative Elements

(in order of decreasing electronegativity)

FONClBrISCH

F	Fluoride
O	Oxygen
N	Nitrogen
Cl	Chlorine
Br	Bromine
I	Iodine
S	Sulfur
C	Carbon
H	Hydroen

Diatomic Elements

FONClBrICH

F	Fluorine
O	Oxygen
N	Nitrogen
Cl	Chlorine
Br	Bromine
I	Iodine
H	Hydrogen

Tip: alternatively, you can use the classic mnemonic: BrINClHOF (pronounced "brinkle-hoff"). Note that these are all the most electronegative elements excluding Sulfur (S)

Strong Acids

SO I Brought NO Clean ClOthes

SO	H_2SO_4
I	HI
Br	HBr
NO	HNO_3
Cl	HCl
ClO	$HClO_4$

Water-Solubility Rules

Always Soluble

NAG-SAG

N	Nitrates (NO_3^-)
A	Acetates ($C_2H_3O_2^-$)
G	Group 1A (Li^+, Na^+, etc.)
S	Sulfates (SO_4^{2-})
A	Ammonium (NH_4^+)
G	Group 7A (F^-, Cl^-, etc.)

Exceptions

Let Me Sit @ Castro's Bar!

L	Lead (Pb2$^+$)	Ca	Ca^{2+}
M	Mercury (Hg2$^+$)	Stro	Sr^{2+} (strontium)
S	Silver (Ag^+)	Ba	Ba^{2+}

Tip: if you like video-games or space, an alternate to NAG-SAG is: GG NASA!... If you like cars, try: GAS GAN. In general, making mnemonics via things you already enjoy or identify with is a great strategy

Redox Reactions

OIL RIG

OIL	Oxidation is Loss (of electrons)
RIG	Reduction is Gain (of electrons)

General Chemistry Notes

General Chemistry Notes

General Chemistry Notes

General Chemistry Notes

General Chemistry Notes

General Chemistry Notes

General Chemistry Notes

Cheat Sheet

General Chemistry

Chapter 3

Organic Chemistry

Isomers

C-SDE

C	Consitutional Isomers
S	Stereoisomers
D	Diastereomers
E	Enantiomers

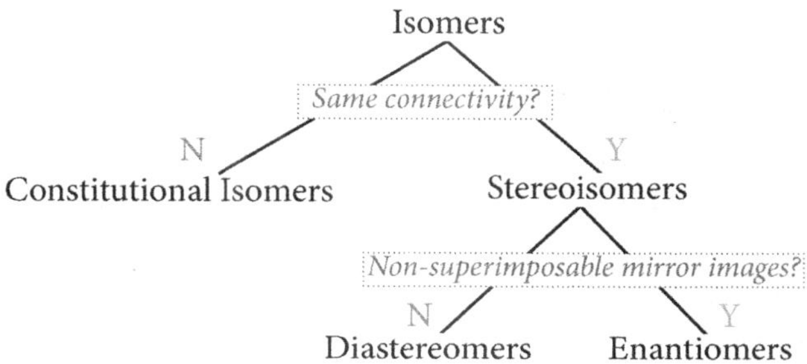

Cis/trans Isomers Nomenclature

ZZE

Z	Zame Zide (cis)
E	Epposite (trans)

Alpha vs. Beta Carbohydrates

If I bow down to Alpha,
you Beta beat me up

Alpha (α) = trans/down

Beta (β) = cis/up

Reaction Types

SEA CAN of PEAs in the MORN

Substitution Electrophilic - Aromatic

Carbonyl - Addition Nucleophillic

Pi bonds - Electrophilic Addition

Most Other Reactions
- Nucleophilic Substitution

Carboxylic Acids

For Ace People Brings Valuable Capital

F	Formic	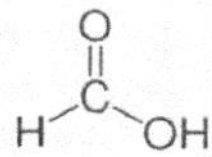
A	Acetic	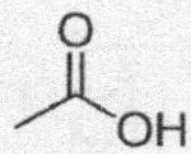
P	Propionic	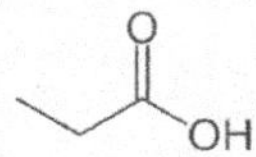
B	Butyric	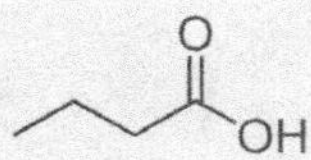
V	Valeric	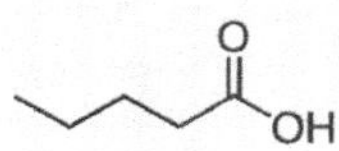
C	Caproic	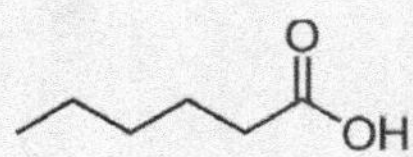

Carbon Chain Prefixes

Me Enjoy Peanut Butter

M	1 Meth-
E	2 Eth-
P	3 Prop-
B	4 But-

Aromatic Substituent Prefixes

Ore More Pore

O	Ortho-
M	Meta-
P	Para-

Spectroscopy and Chromatography

Thin Layer Chromatography Plate

Polar bears are lower and slower

On problems with a TLC plate, polar compounds move more slowly up the plate (lower R_f value) than non-polar compounds (higher R_f value).

NMR Spectroscopy

De-shield is down-field

De-shielded signals are more down-field ie. have higher ppm values. There is less shielding as a result of decreasing electron density around a nucleus or nuclei. Thus the magnetic field from the electrons is being overpowered by the NMR's external magnetic field. The protons need a higher frequency to achieve resonance, thus moving them down-field.

L Amino Acids vs. D Carbohydrates

Los Angeles vs. District of Columbia

LA = L Amino Acids

DC = D Carbohydrates

4 Factors of Molecule Stability

Stable RISE

R	Resonance
I	Induction
S	Size
E	Electronegativity *ie. minimizing charge*

Adding Amine to Carbonyl Group

SE PI

SE	Secondary amine = Enamine
PI	Primary amine = Imine

Note: tertiary and quaternary amines don't react with the C=0 group

Reducing Agents

Reduce NaAKed LiCE

NaAK	$NaBH_4$ = Aldehydes & Ketones
LiCE	$LiAlH_4$ = Carboxylic acid & Esters

Meta-directing Groups on Benzene Rings

Queen Elizabeth's Second Navy
Commands, Controls, Communicates

Q	Quaternary amino $-NR_3^+$
E	Ester -COOR
S	Sulfonic Acid $-SO_3H$
N	Nitro $-NO_2$
C	Carbonyl -CHO
C	Carboxyl -COOH
C	Cyano -CN

Ortho- and Para-directing Groups on Benzene Rings

AHA AHA Phil

A	Alkyl -R
H	Halogen -X
A	Alkoxyl -OR
A	Amino (all except $-NR_3^+$) $-NH_2$ -NHR $-NR_2$
H	Hydroxyl -OH
A	Amide -NHCOR
P	Phenyl $-C_6H_5$

Organic Chemistry Notes

Organic Chemistry Notes

Organic Chemistry Notes

Organic Chemistry Notes

Organic Chemistry Notes

Organic Chemistry Notes

Organic Chemistry Notes

Cheat Sheet

Organic Chemistry

Chapter 4

Physics

Electromagnetic Waves

Rich Men Invented Very Unusual X-ray Guns

R	Radio waves
M	Microwaves
I	Infrared
V	Visible light
U	Ultraviolet
X	X-Rays
G	Gamma Rays

Tip: An alternative mnemonic if you prefer: Raging Martians Invade Venus Using X-ray Guns

Metric System

Kings Hate Dragons Because
Dragons Can't Make Microscopes

K	Kilo-
H	Hector-
D	Deca-
B	Base-
D	Deci-
C	Centi-
M	Milli-
M	Micro-

Equations

Power

♪ Twinkle twinkle little star,
power equals I squared R

$P = I^2R$ (or $P = V^2/R$, $P = IV$)

Gibb's Free Energy

Gibby Hates Tartar Sauce

$\Delta G = \Delta H - T\Delta S$

Heat

Q equals MCAT!

$Q = mC\Delta T$

Electrostatic Equations

Frick U Evil Vampires!

$F_E = kqq / r^2$ Electrostatic Force	$U_E = kqq / r$ Electrostatic Potential
$E = kq / r^2$ Electric Field Strength	$V = kq / r$ Voltage/Potential

Lenses

The IRS gave me UVB sun cancer

IRS	Inverted, real, smaller (coming toward 2*f*)
UVB	Upright, virtual, bigger (as it gets closer than *f*... it burns!)

Tip: An alternative mnemonic: FIG PB ("Fig Peanut Butter"). Use if you prefer

Capacitive and Inductive Circuits

ELI the ICE man

The EMF (E) for an inductive (L) circuit is greater than the current (I) While the current (I) for a capacitive circuit (C) is greater than the EMF (E).

Physics Notes

Physics Notes

Physics Notes

Physics Notes

Physics Notes

Physics Notes

Physics Notes

Cheat Sheet

Physics

Chapter 5

Biology

Cell Cycle

Go Sally! Go Make Children!

G	Growth Phase 1
S	S phase *(DNA synthesis/replication)*
G	Growth Phase 2
M	Mitosis
C	Cytokinesis

Cell Division

Pee MAT

P	Prophase
M	Metaphase
A	Anaphase
T	Telophase (+cytokinesis)

Taxonomy

King Phillip Came For Gold & Silver

K	Kingdom
P	Phylum
C	Class Order
F	Family
G	Genus
S	Species

Kingdoms

FM APP

F	Fungi
M	Monera
A	Animals
P	Plants
P	Protista

Gastrointestinal Hormones

Garlic Cloves Smell Exquisite

G	Gastrin
C	Cholecystokinin
S	Secretin
E	Enterogastrone

Pancreas Hormones

Something's In the Glue!

S	Somastatin
I	Insulin
G	Glucagon

Anterior Pituitary Hormones

FLAT PEG

F	Follicle-stimulating (FSH)
L	Luteinizing (LH)
A	Adrenocorticotropic (ACTH)
T	Thyroid stimulating (TSH)
P	Prolactin
E	Endorphins
G	Growth hormone (GH)

Calcium Hormones

Calciton*in*, Parathy*rid*

Calcitonin = Calcium IN

Parathyroid = RIDs Calcium

Hormones ↑ Blood Glucose

GG NETS

G	Glucagon
G	Glucocorticosteroids
N	Norepinephrine
E	Epinephrine
T	Thyroid Hormones *(thyroxine and triiodothyronine)*
S	Somatotropin

Causes of Deviation from Hardy-Weinberg Equilibrium

Mutant Michaela Does Not Smoke

M	Mutations
M	Migration
D	Drift
N	Non-random Mating
S	Selection

Pancreas Secretion

BAD PIGS

B	Beta-cells
A	Alpha-cells
D	Delta-cells
P	(of the) Pancreas
I	(secrete) Insulin
G	Glucagon
S	Somatostatin

Fat Soluble Vitamins

Vitamin D-A-K-E

Tip: try to use this mnemonic as in other versions you may confuse Vitamin K with Vitamin C due to the pronunciation

White Blood Cells

(in order of highest frequency)

Nobody Likes My Educational Background?

N	Neutrophils
L	Lymphocytes
M	Monocytes
E	Eosinophils
B	Basophils

Tip: ***Note that granulocytes end in -phil and agranulocytes end in -cyt**e*. A good mnemonic for remembering granulocytes is: "Gruncle BEN", ie. Granulocytes = Basiophil, Eosinophil, Neutrophil

Immunoglobulins

MADGE

IgM

IgA

IgD

IgG

IgE

MHC Class I vs. II

MHC ONE, you're DONE. MHC TWO, I help YOU

Major histocompatibility complex, or MHC, are membrane-bound proteins that display or present antigens for T-cells. MHC I recruits killer T-cells (your done), while MHC II recruits helper T-cells (I help you). Note that MHC I will display antigens from intracellular pathogens (viruses/bacteria), while MHC II from extracellular pathogens. Antigen Presenting cells (APCs) like macrophages, dendritic cells, and B-cells always have MHC II.

Skeletal Muscle Sarcomere Contraction

HAIZ (haze) that muscle!

H	H-zone
A	A-band
I	I-band
Z	Z-line

Ciliary Muscle Contraction

Close Causes Ciliary Contraction

Close objects cause the Ciliary muscles to contract, causing the zonular fibres to decrease tension. This causes the lens to take on a "fatter" or more spherical shape, which allows greater focusing power on the (close) image, allowing the vertex distance to decrease to land perfectly at the fovea for photo-receptors.

Intestine Parts

(in order)

Dow Jones Industrial ACCoRd

Small Intestine

D	Duodenum
J	Jejunum
I	Ileum

Large Intestine

A	Appendix
C	Cecum
C	Colon
R	Rectum

Epidermal Layers

Come Let's Get SunBurnt

C	Stratum corneum
L	Stratum lucidum
G	Stratum granulosum
S	Stratum spinosum
B	Stratum basale

Below these are the basement membrane, which supports the epidermis and endothelial tissue attached, as well as being a diffusion barrier to the dermis just below.

7 Pathway of Sperm

SEVEn UP

S	Seminiferous tubules
E	Epididymis
V	Vas deferens
E	Ejaculatory duct
U	Urethra
P	Penis

Fetal Development Stages

Many Babies Get Naps

M	Morula (after fertilization → 1, 2, 4, 8)
B	Blastula (looks blasted out bc. of hollow cavity: blastocoel)
G	Gastrula
N	Neuralation

Chordate Traits

Do Not Pinch People

D	Dorsal Nerve Cord
N	Notochord
P	Pharyngeal Slits
P	Post-anal Tail

Neuron

Dangerous MASS Nervousness

D	Dendrites
M	Myelin Sheath
A	Axon
S	Synapse + synaptic vesicles
S	Soma
N	Nodes of Ranvier

Tip: Another simple trick is to remember that the neuron is a salty banana: theres a bunch of Na+ on the outside, and K+ on the inside (ie. at resting membrane potential). Another specific mnemonic: 321Nokia, for 3 Na+ Out, 2 K- In, 1 ATP used

Microtubule Movements

DRAKe

D	Dynein
R	Retrograde (backward)
A	Anterograde (forward)
K	Kinesin

Dynein is a motor protein that drives cargo toward the minus end of the microtubule. Kinesin is a motor protein that moves toward the plus end. Eg. in neuron axonal transport, soma→axon terminal = dynein, and axon terminal→soma = kinesin.

Sympathetic vs. Parasympathetic

Fight or Flight vs. Rest and Digest

Another way to understand this: the prefix para- comes from Greek and means "alongside". Thus, someone standing alongside you or guiding you would make you feel calmer. On the other hand, if you saw that person running away, you would panic.

Nerve Fibers and Location in Spinal Cord

SAME DAVE

SA	Sensory = afferent
ME	Motor = efferent
DA	Dorsal = afferent (back)
VE	Ventral = efferent (front)

Brain Lobes

Tear Freud's Pants Off!

T	Temporal
F	Frontal
P	Parietal
O	Occipital

Limbic System

HATCH

H	Hippocampus
A	Amygdala
T	Thalamus
C	Cerebellum
H	Hypothalamus

Brain Stem

Pavlov's Really Frickin' Mad!

P	Pons
RF	Reticular Formation
M	Medulla

+ Cerebellum = Hindbrain

Neurotransmitters

DASE or SADE (famous singer)

D	Dopamine
A	Acetylcholine
S	Seratonin
E	Endorphins

Functions of Meninges

RAP

R	Reabsorb CSF
A	Anchor brain
P	Protect brain

Meninges Layers

PAD

P	Pia mater
A	Arachnoid space
D	Dura mater

Parkinson's Disease Symptoms

Patients feel in a TRAP

T	Tremor at rest
R	Plants
A	Akinesia *(a- = without; kin- = movement)*
F	Posture stooped

PD is a progressive nervous system disorder that appears primarily between the ages of 50 and 60 and is characterized by the loss of dopaminergic neurons within the substantia nigra pars compacta of the basal ganglia. The first signs of the diseasetypically manifest as a hand tremor. As the disease progresses, the symptoms intensify. In the later stages of Parkinson's, behavioral problems and dementia surface, making normal living difficult.

Cardiac Conduction System

Stab A BaBy Puppy

S	SA Node
A	AV Node
B	Bundle of HIS
B	Bundle branches
P	Purkinje fibers

The SA node starts the conduction sequence by causing the atrial muscles to contract. Then, the signal travels to the AV node, then through the bundle of HIS, down the bundle branches, and then through the Purkinje fibers, causing the ventricles to contract. This signal generates an electrical current that can be seen on an electrocardiogram, or EKG.

Atrioventricular Valves

LAB RAT

LEFT Atrioventricular **BICUSPID**

RIGHT Atrioventricular **TRICUSPID**

Biology Notes

Biology Notes

Biology Notes

Biology Notes

Biology Notes

Biology Notes

Biology Notes

Biology Notes

Biology Notes

Cheat Sheet

Biology

Chapter 6

Biochemistry

Enzyme Types

LIL HOT

L	Ligases ("synthases") $A + B \rightleftarrows A\text{-}B$
I	Isomerases $A \rightleftarrows \text{Iso-}A$
L	Ligases ("synthetases") $A + B + XTP \rightleftarrows A\text{-}B + XDP$ *(X = A, G, U, C)*
H	Hydrolases $A\text{-}B + H_2O \rightleftarrows A\text{-}H + B\text{-}OH$
O	Oxidoreductases $A_{red} + B_{ox} \rightleftarrows A_{ox} + B_{red}$
T	Transferases $A\text{-}B + C \rightleftarrows A + B\text{-}C$

Non-Polar Amino Acids

The Little VAMP PIG

T	Tryptophan
L	Leucine
V	Valine
A	Alanine
M	Methionine
P	Proline
P	Phenylalanine
I	Isoleucine
G	Glycine

Polar Uncharged Amino Acids

Grandma Says Take Care Always

G	Glutamine (Gln)
S	Serine (Aer)
T	Threonine (Thr)
C	Cysteine (Cys)
A	Asparagine (Asn)

Charged Amino Acids

At the GAH-LA

G	Glutamic Acid (Glu)
A	Arginine (Arg)
H	Histidine (His)
L	Lysine (Lys)
A	Aspartic acid (Asp)

Note that negatively charged aspartic acid (Asp) and glutamic acid (Glu) have acidic side chains at neutral ph (7). While the remaining are positively charged with basic side chains.

Positive Amino Acids

HoLA!

H	Histidine
L	Lysine
A	Arginine

These are positively charged at pH=7. Negatively charged ones are aspartic acid (Asp, D) and glutamic acid (Glu, E).

Aromatic Amino Acids

Three Tall Pickles

T	Tyrosine
T	Tryptophan
P	Phenylalanine

Polar (Hydrophilic) Amino Acids

LAH-dy GAGA

L	Lysine
A	Arginine
H	Histidine
G	Glutamate
A	Aspartate
G	Glutamine
A	Asparagine

Glucogenic vs. Ketogenic Amino Acids

TIP That Tractor

T	Tryptophan
I	Isoleucine
P	Phenylalanine
T	Tyrosine
T	Threonine

The above amino acids are **glucogenic AND ketogenic**. There are only 2 only ketogenic: lysine and leucine (only ones that start with L) which means that they can be metabolized into acetyl coA. All remaining amino acids are only glucogenic ie. convertible to glucose via gluconeogenesis: Alanine, arginine, asparagine, aspartate, cysteine, glutamine, glutamate, glycine, histidine, and methionine

Tip: Another simple mnemonic for the above: PIT3 (three Ts)

Hydrophobic Alkyl Side Chains

Very PAIL and scared!

V	Valine
P	Phenylalanine
A	Alanine
I	Isoleucine
L	Leucine

Hydrophobic alkyl side chains are very pale and scared of water ie. hydrophobic.

Molecules in the TCA Cycle

Cuddly Kangaroos Swallow Sweet Fruit, Mumbling Occasionally

C	Citrate
K	Ketoglutarate
S	Succinyl-CoA
S	Succinate
F	Fumarate
M	Malate
O	Oxaloacetate

Tip: Another simple mnemonic for the above: "Can I Keep Selling Shells For Money, Officer?"

Enzymes in the TCA cycle

The Cat CIA Strikes Silently, Frequently Meowing

C	Citrate synthase
C	Cis-aconitase
I	Isocitrate dehydrogenase
A	A-α-ketoglutarate dehydrogenase
S	Succinyl CoA synthetase
S	Succinate dehydrogenase
F	Fumarase
M	Malate dehydrogenase

TCA Cycle Products

FAD got kicked in the (3) 'NADs, Get The Paramedic!

FAD	+3 NADH
NAD	+1 FADH2
GTP	+1 GTP

Molecules in Glycolysis

Good God Father Frank! Don't Go Buy
Pricey Pepsi Pop Please

G	Glucose
G	Glucose-6-phosphate
F	Fructose-6-phosphate
F	Fructose-1,6-bisphosphate
D	DHAP
G	Glyceraldehyde-3-phosphate
B	1, 3-bisphosphoglycerate
P	3-phosphoglycerate
P	2-phosphoglycerate
P	Phosphoenolpyruvate (PEP)
P	Pyruvate

Enzymes in Irreversible Steps of Glycolysis

He Gobbles Pot Pie Keenly

H	Hexokinase
G	Glucokinase
P	PFK-1
P	Pyruvate
K	Kinase

B Vitamins

That Red Ninja Pierced Pablo Before Frolicking (Cy)Silently

B1	**T**	Thiamine
B2	**R**	Riboflavin
B3	**N**	Niacin
B5	**P**	Pantothenic acid
B6	**P**	Pyridoxal phosphate
B7	**B**	Biotin
B9	**F**	Folic acid
B12	**C**	Cyanocobalamin

Pyrimidines / Purines

CUT the Py

C	Cytosine
U	Uracil
T	Thiamine

Pur(e) As Gold

A	Adenine
G	Guanine

Adenine bonds to Thymine; Cytosine bonds to Guanine. A good mnemonic for this relationship is: "Aye Thy Cy Guy"

Stop Codons

U Are Annoying, U Go Away, U Are Gone

UAA

UGA

UAG

Start codon: AUG ("Are U Going?")

Types of Blots

S D
N R
o o
W P

S	Southern Blot = DNA	D
N	Northern Blot = RNA	R
W	Western Blot = Proteins	P

Biochemistry Notes

Biochemistry Notes

Biochemistry Notes

Biochemistry Notes

Biochemistry Notes

Biochemistry Notes

Biochemistry Notes

Biochemistry Notes

✎ Cheat Sheet

Biochemistry

Chapter 7

Psychology

Freud's Stages of Psycho-sexual Development

Old Aged People Love Grandchildren

O	Oral Stage
A	Anal Stage
P	Phallic Stage
L	Latent Stage
G	Genital Stage

Piaget's Stages of Cognitive Development

Some People Can Fly

S	Sensorimotor
P	Pre-operational
C	Concrete Operational
F	Formal Operational

Erikson's Psychosocial Development Stages

Trust the Auto Insurance Industry, and Identify Intimately Geniuses with Integrity

Trust	Trust vs. Mistrust	0-1
Auto...	Autonomy vs. Shame and Doubt	1-3
In...	Initiative vs. Guilt	3-6
Industry	Industry vs. Inferiority	6-12
Identi...	Identity vs. Confusion	12-20
Intimate	Intimacy vs. Isolation	20-40
Gen...	Generativity vs. Stagnation	40-65
Integrity	Integrity vs. Despair	65+

This mnemonic still requires you to drill the entire conflict and what age it is associated with (the right column... For ranges all you need to memorize the first number in each range, 0, 1, 3, 6, etc.). This is important as it is how the concept will be tested on the MCAT.

Tip: If strapped for time, internalize another simpler, albeit more reductive mnemonic is: TAI4GI (pronounced "tie for guy") . Each letter corresponds to a stage, with "I4" referring to the 4 instances of stages starting with I (drill these)

Kohlberg's Moral Stages

PS. Good Luck SUE!

PS	Punishment avoidance & Self-interest *preconventional stage*
GL	"Good boy" & Law and order *conventional stage*
SUE	Social contract & Universal Ethics Principles *postconventional stage*

Kubler-Ross Stages of Grief

Death Always Brings Definite Acceptance

D	Denial
A	Anger
B	Bargaining
D	Depression
A	Acceptance

Bandura's Social Cognitive Theory

AM I Motivated?

A	Attention
M	Memory = Retention
I	Imitation = Motor Reproduction
M	Motivation

Bandura's social cognitive, or social learning theory highlights the role of self-belief in human cognition. With this he believed individuals could overcome their human sense of "failing" and dysfunction through this framework of controlling ones thoughts, feelings, and actions. For example, if a teacher is positive and verbally encourages students during tasks, students build self-belief and self-efficacy to succeed in performing tasks via observation and modeling despite possible setbacks or different situations/contexts.

Types of Reinforcement

People Need Proper Care

P	Positive
N	Negative
P	Primary
C	Conditional

Theories of Personality

Behave Psycho Human! Try Socializing!

B	Behaviorism
P	Psychoanalytic
H	Humanistic
T	Trait
S	Social/Cognitive

Theories of Emotion

Schacter-Singer Theory: A + A = E

A	Arousal
A	Appraisal
E	Emotions

James-Lange Theory: E→A→R

E	Event
A	Arousal
R	Response

Cannon-Bard Theory: ABC

A	Arousal
B	Brain
C	Concurrent

3 Components of Parallel Processing

Crayons Make Shapes

C	Color
M	Motion
S	Shapes

3 Components of Attitude

ABC

A	Affective
B	Behavioral
C	Cognitive

5 Elements of Personality

OCEAN

O	Openness
C	Conscientiousness
E	Extraversion
A	Agreeableness
N	Neuroticism

Tip: alternatively you can use the mnemonic CANOE, depending on your preference.

3 Most Important Features of Attraction

Special Relationship with Partner

S	Similarity
R	Reciprocity
P	Proximity

Most Common Mental and Psychiatric Disorders

Dad And Brother Protect And Serve

D	Depression
A	Anxiety
B	Bipolar Disorder
P	Phobia
A	Autism
S	Schizophrenia

Tip: A simpler mnemonic you can use is: DABnPAS (pronounced "dab and pass")

Major Depressive Disorder Symptoms

Can All Individuals Go Everywhere Without Shoes?

Loss of:

C	Concentration
A	Appetite
I	Interest
G	Guilt
E	Energy
W	Will to Live
S	Sleep

Frontal Lobe Functions

SLIME

S	Speech Production
L	Long-Term Planning
I	Impulse Control
M	Motor Fuction
E	Executive Function

Temporal Lobe Functions

MESS

M	Memory
E	Emotion
S	Speech Processing (Wernicke's)
S	Sound Perception

Self-determination Theory Components

CAR

C	Competence
A	Autonomy
R	Relatedness

4 Primary Factors of Motivation

Does Anyone Need Ice?

D	Drives
A	Arousal
N	Needs
I	Instincts

Tip: an alternative mnemonic is "DANI is motivated". Use this if you tend to remember names well or prefer it

General Adaptation Syndrome (GAS) Components

ARE you GASsy?

A	Alarm
R	Resistance
E	Exhaustion

4 Ethical Tenets

wanNA JoB?

N	Non-maleficence
A	Autonomy
J	Justice
B	Beneficence

Tip: A simpler alternative mnemonic is "BANJo", if you prefer

Brain Waves

(Sequential Order)

BATs Drink Blood

B	Beta (awake)
A	Alpha (drowsy; N1)
T	Theta (no enviro. awareness; sleep spindles; K-complexes; N2)
D	Delta (N3+4)
B	Beta (return back for REM)

On the MCAT, you might need to associate wave types with sleep stages and cycle order and associated info. (eg. delta is associated with sleep stage N3: deep sleep, where parasomnias like sleepwalking can occur)

4 Primary Stimuli

Cute Puppies Love Toys

C	Chemical
P	Pressure
L	Light
T	Temperature

6 Universal Emotions

ASDFGH
(row on keyboard)

A	Anger
S	Surprise
D	Disgust
F	Fear
G	Gloomy (Sadness)
H	Happiness

An alternate mnemonic: All Humans Feel Da Same Sh**

Tip: take a study break and watch Pixar movie Inside Out! Each character represents each of Ekman's emotions. Although, the director and writers decided to omit one... surprise!

Types of Stressors

NEED

N	Nutritional
E	Environmental
E	Emotional
D	Dental

Physiological Markers of Emotions

PART B

Changes in:

P	Pulse
A	Adrenaline
R	Respiration rate
T	Temperature
B	Blood pressure

Maslow's Hierarchy of Needs

Please Stop Liking Stupid Sh**

P	Physiological
S	Safety
L	Love
S	Self-esteem
S	Self-actualization

Psychology Notes

Psychology Notes

Psychology Notes

Psychology Notes

Psychology Notes

Psychology Notes

Psychology Notes

Psychology Notes

Psychology Notes

Cheat Sheet

Psychology

Chapter 8

Sociology

7 Identity Types

RC GRASP

R	Race/Ethnicity
C	Class
G	Gender
R	Religion
A	Age
S	Sexual Orientation
P	Politics

Social Facilitation Theoretical Approaches

Always Eat Strawberries And Spinach

A	Activation Theory
E	Evaluation Approach
S	Social Interaction Theory
A	Attention Approach
G	Self-Presentation Approach

Tip: An alternative mnemonic is "AT the SPA, SIT, pay attention and evaluate". This can be useful as it triggers location-based and spatial memory

Social Norm Types

Provolone DIPS

P	Proscriptive
D	Descriptive
I	Injunctive
P	Prescriptive
S	Subjective

7 Agents of Socialization

Find Peers Who Graduate Medical School Rapidly

F	Family
P	Peers
W	Workplace
G	Government
M	Mass Media
S	School
R	Religion

7 Elements of Culture

VAN-LESS

V	Values
A	Artifacts
N	Norms
L	Language
E	Economy
S	Symbols
S	Society

6 Factors of Globalization

Pumpkin THIEF!

P	Politics
T	Technology
H	Historical
I	Industrial Organization
E	Economy
F	Financial

5 Characteristics of an Ideal Bureaucracy

Well Formed Hierarchy Divides Impartially

W	Well-trained Employees
F	Formalized Rules
H	Hierarchy of Organization
D	Division of Labor
I	Impartiality

5 Types of Non-Verbal Communication

I Get Free Body Pillows

I	Eye Contact
G	Gestures
F	Facial Expressions
B	Body Language
P	Posture

Tip: An alternative mnemonic: FIG PB ("Fig Peanut Butter"). Use if you prefer

Sociology Notes

Sociology Notes

Sociology Notes

Sociology Notes

Sociology Notes

Sociology Notes

Sociology Notes

Cheat Sheet

Sociology

Made in the USA
Monee, IL
13 September 2026

62981873R00118